'To ensure that cardiac patients receive the best possible care during the worst possible times' - Adrian Levine & Joel Dunning

We are greatly indebted to the many hours of work put into the
creation of this course and this handbook by many clinicians including :
Christian Karcher, Adrian Levine, George Zhou, Alex Yartsev, David McCormack,
Amy Rogers, Craig Jurisevic

Table of Contents

CALS around the world

In 2003 in Blackpool, United Kingdom, a patient 4 hours post cardiac surgery had a cardiac arrest. Over the following four hours his chest was re-opened three times and eventually the patient was re-grafted in his Intensive Care Unit (ICU) bed on bypass.

Many of the nursing and junior medical staff reported they felt disorganised, were of little help to the situation and would have performed much better if they had a defined and well-practised role. In response to this we created the Cardiac Surgery Advanced Life Support Course.

We have devised a set of protocols that address the management of a patient suffering a cardiac arrest following cardiac surgery, and all common serious complications in ICU or on the ward. Our aim was to create a common language for all clinicians looking after patients post-cardiothoracic surgery.

This protocol has grown and has been accepted as the official protocol of the European Association of Cardiothoracic Surgery and the European Resuscitation Council.

The Society of Thoracic Surgery also created an expert consensus statement which is published in the Annals of Thoracic surgery (March 2017) and sets these protocols as the standard of care in the USA.

In Australasia, the CALS-ANZ steering group created guidelines for Cardiothoracic Advanced Life Support which have been endorsed by the Australian & New Zealand Society Of Cardiac and Thoracic Surgeons (ANZSCTS), and the Australian and New Zealand Intensive Care Society (ANZICS) in 2020.

We hope this course will provide you with knowledge, skills and confidence to apply validated protocols in the treatment of deteriorating cardiothoracic patients.

Joel Dunning and Adrian Levine

Founders of CALS

Background

Every year more than 15,000 patients undergo cardiac surgery in Australia and New Zealand. The incidence of cardiac arrest after cardiac surgery is between 0.7 and 5.2% depending on the procedure performed. As a rule of thumb, the more complex the procedure, the higher the risk of complications, including cardiac arrest.

The majority of cardiac arrests occur within 24 hours of surgery with approximately half of them occurring in the first 3 hours after the operation. Reassuringly, survival in this patient population is high compared to other in-hospital arrests (75 vs 39%). The reasons for this include prompt recognition and treatment of the deterioration due to the high level of monitoring in the ICU, a high proportion of reversible causes, and the proven benefits of early resternotomy, internal cardiac massage and internal defibrillation. Ventricular fibrillation (VF) is the cause of cardiac arrest in 25-50% of cases, and in the intensive care unit setting this can be immediately identified and treated. Cardiac tamponade and major bleeding account for a large percentage of the remaining causes of arrests. Both conditions can be quickly relieved by prompt resuscitation and emergency resternotomy, to relieve tamponade and control bleeding.

Prompt recognition and treatment by ICU staff improves survival. Practising protocol-based arrest management has been shown to reduce by 50% the time to chest reopening and reduce complications resulting from the resternotomy after cardiac surgery.

The application of standard ALS protocols in post-surgical cardiothoracic patients may lead to avoidable adverse events as and hence specific resuscitation protocols have been developed and established in Europe, North America and Australasia.

The Australian and New Zealand Resuscitation Council (ANZCOR) issued its latest guideline on resuscitation in special circumstances in November 2011 providing basic recommendations for the resuscitation of patients after cardiac surgery. These guidelines acknowledge a potential risk of external chest compressions in patients after cardiac surgery and recommend a re-sternotomy in adequately staffed and equipped ICUs. Subsequently, the American Society of Thoracic Surgeons (STS) published their Expert Consensus Guidelines in 2017.

These documents have prompted many clinicians managing cardiac surgical patients to evaluate more carefully how cardiac arrests are managed in their own units. There is now widespread recognition that a cardiac arrest after cardiac surgery is sufficiently different to warrant a distinct treatment algorithm in order to optimise survival after arrest in this group of patients.

In 2017, the Australasian steering committee for CALS (CALS-ANZ) was formed with the Royal Melbourne Hospital becoming the first Centre of Excellence for CALS training in Australasia. Subsequently, CALS-ANZ developed local guidelines for the management of cardiothoracic emergencies, which form the basis of this handbook.

CALS ANZ Guidelines

The Australasian CALS guidelines are based on a consensus established amongst senior clinicians in Australia and New Zealand and have been endorsed by the Australian and New Zealand Society of Cardiac and Thoracic Surgeons (ANZSCTS) and the Australian and New Zealand Intensive Care Society (ANZICS).

The guidelines were developed using a Delphi consensus as well as a systematic literature review. The Delphi survey expert panel consisted of 79 specialists in the fields of Intensive Care, Cardiac Anaesthesia and Cardiac surgery from Australia and New Zealand.

The CALS protocol addresses many issues unique to the cardiac surgical patient including the timing of emergency resternotomy, the number of attempts at defibrillation before resternotomy, the administration of adrenaline, ventilator management, infusion and pacemaker settings, emergency resternotomy instrumentation sets, and cardiac arrests presenting in the non-ICU setting and under special circumstances.

This protocol applies to all cardiothoracic patients in the ICU including paediatric, minimally invasive cardiac surgical (with limitations), LVAD and transplant patients.

The CALS-ANZ arrest algorithm

Cardiac arrests in a monitored environment such as an ICU can be diagnosed instantaneously by loss of pulsatility in all invasive pressures (arterial, pulmonary arterial, central venous) as well as loss of pulsatility on plethysmography. In ventilated patients a marked drop in end-tidal CO_2 is observed.

The CALS-ANZ algorithm begins with an assessment of the patient's rhythm and has three distinct treatment pathways:

1) If the patient is in pulseless ventricular tachycardia (VT) or ventricular fibrillation (VF) cardiac arrest, adhesive defibrillator pads are attached and up to three stacked shocks are delivered.

2) If the patient is in asystole or severe bradycardia with epicardial pacing wires in place, the patient is paced in DOO mode.

3) If the patient is in pulseless electrical activity (PEA) arrest and is paced the time of the arrest, the pacemaker is briefly paused to exclude underlying VF (which would require defibrillation)

During this initial phase of assessment and management, external chest compressions may be withheld for up to 60 seconds in an attempt to immediately reverse the cardiac arrest by either defibrillation or pacing following the CALS-ANZ algorithm. The rationale for this is as follows:

- External cardiac massage carries a significant risk of trauma to thoracic structures in the early post-operative phase after cardiac surgery.

- Of the possible causes of cardiac arrest after cardiac surgery, two (asystole or shockable rhythms) can be reversed immediately by pacing or defibrillation.

- For PEA after cardiac surgery, the major causes (pericardial tamponade, tension pneumothorax and massive haemorrhage) render external chest compressions potentially ineffective, insofar as they are unlikely to lead to sufficient cardiac output or brain perfusion.

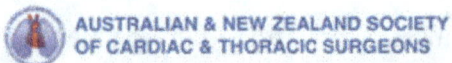 AUSTRALIAN & NEW ZEALAND SOCIETY OF CARDIAC & THORACIC SURGEONS

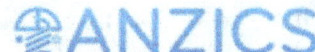 ANZICS

CARDIAC ARREST

ASSESS AND MANAGE RHYTHM

VF or VT	ASYSTOLE SEVERE BRADY	PEA
3 stacked shocks	pace - if wires available	pause pacing to exclude underlying VF

START EXTERNAL CHEST COMPRESSIONS
AND
START EMERGENCY RESTERNOTOMY
AIM OPEN CHEST <5MIN FROM ARREST

Continue CPR with single DCR shocks until resternotomy	Continue CPR until resternotomy	Continue CPR until resternotomy
300mg Amiodarone (iv)	Consider external pacing	

Change from ventilator to BMV
Increase FiO2 to 1.0. verify ETT patency
Ensure bilateral air entry
Do not give Adrenaline unless a senior clinician. experienced in CALS advises this
Do not delay basic life support by more than 60sec.

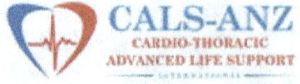 CALS-ANZ CARDIO-THORACIC ADVANCED LIFE SUPPORT

Emergency resternotomy

If the above measures fail to establish return of spontaneous circulation, a resternotomy must be performed. In order to reduce any delays in reopening the chest, preparation for emergency resternotomy should commence immediately at the time of the arrest, including two or three staff members putting on sterile gowns and gloves and preparing the emergency resternotomy set.

The emergency resternotomy is an integral part of the CALS arrest management for all patients within 10 days of their last operation. Beyond the 10th post-operative day, a senior clinician should decide whether emergency resternotomy is to be performed.

Resternotomy procedure

The technique of emergency resternotomy is described in greater detail in Chapter 8.

After removing the sternotomy dressing, a one-piece adhesive surgical drape is placed on the patient's chest without prior skin prep. A short period of 'sterile' external cardiac massage may be required until all of the resternotomy equipment is ready.

After cutting skin sutures and removal of sternal closure devices (wires, plates, cables) a retractor is inserted to allow for exposure of the heart. The pericardium may have to be reopened if it is closed. Chest reopening should be completed within 5 minutes from the onset of circulatory arrest. Any blood clots are carefully removed, internal cardiac massage is commenced using the two-handed technique and, if in a shockable rhythm, the heart is defibrillated with 20 joules using internal defibrillator pads.

Teamwork and communication

Effective teamwork is an essential component of successful emergency management.

The CALS-ANZ protocol defines clear role allocations and each of those roles should be taken by an appropriately trained team member. Individual roles and teamwork should be regularly practised in interprofessional and interdisciplinary simulation training. Chapter 6 (Human Factors) addresses those aspects in detail.

Airway Management

The CALS-ANZ guidelines recommend standard principles to address any problems related to the patient's airway or ventilation. If the patient is not intubated at the time of the cardiac arrest, ventilation should initially be performed via bag-mask-ventilation or a supraglottic airway with an FiO2 of 1.0. Endotracheal intubation should not delay attempts to address reversible causes nor chest reopening and is best performed once the resternotomy is completed or return of spontaneous circulation (ROSC) is restored.

Drugs and infusions

Cardiac arrests in patients after cardiac surgery are often quickly reversible and circulating standard ALS doses of adrenaline (i.e. 1mg i.v.) can therefore cause excessive hypertension and arrhythmias when achieving ROSC. Therefore, only small doses of adrenaline (eg 50-100 micrograms i.v.) should be given. Amiodarone should be considered for refractory shockable rhythms.

Since drug errors, adverse reactions and inadvertent bolus administration of vasodilatory drugs (e.g. sedatives and analgesics) may precipitate a cardiac arrest, all pre-arrest infusions should be paused and checked for errors.

Cardiovascular Physiology

In order to optimise the circulation of a postoperative cardiac patient, it is important to understand the underlying cardiovascular physiological principles. The goal of post cardiac surgery cardiovascular optimisation is to maintain tissue perfusion for all organs while the heart recovers. Successful tissue perfusion can be demonstrated by normal end-organ function (kidney function and urine output, normal liver function, cognitive ability, adequate oxygenation) and the absence of lactate accumulation on blood gas testing.

Cardiac Output

Cardiac output is a function of heart rate and stroke volume.

Cardiac Output = Heart Rate x Stroke Volume

The optimal heart rate for an adult is around 80-100/min. Although a low cardiac output in the context of bradycardia can be improved by pacing the heart, it is important to understand that a very fast heart rate (e.g atrial tachycardia or rapid atrial fibrillation) will lead to a decreased cardiac output as a result of decreased duration of diastole.

In addition to the optimal heart rate, sinus rhythm maximises cardiac output as atrial contraction contributes to about 20% of the stroke volume.

Stroke volume is influenced by three factors: preload, contractility and afterload.

Preload is the stretching of the myocardial cells just before contraction and refers most commonly to the end-diastolic volume. There is compelling evidence that static pressures such as the central venous pressure (CVP) and the left ventricular end-diastolic pressure (LVEDP or wedge pressure) are inadequate markers of preload and there is a movement towards dynamic markers. Preload can be optimised by ensuring sufficient filling of the ventricle. Fluid loading will, up to a certain point, improve contractility by optimising the Frank-Starling curve. Beyond that optimal filling point however, additional fluid loading may lead to overstretching of the myocardial cells and contribute to heart failure.

Contractility refers to the force with which the myocardial cells can shorten (contract) and is influenced (as described above) by preload and also the effects of beta-adrenergic catecholamines such as dobutamine and adrenaline.

Afterload is considered the resistance against which the ventricles eject and is closely related to the pulmonary artery pressure and aorta pressure respectively. A reduction of afterload leads to an increased stroke volume and vice versa.

Oxygen delivery (DO_2)

Adequate delivery of oxygen to the peripheral tissues and organs is the ultimate aim of optimising the cardio-respiratory system.

Oxygen delivery is a function of cardiac output and oxygen content (CaO_2), that is the sum of the oxygen bound to haemoglobin and dissolved in plasma.

DO2 = CO x CaO_2

Blood Pressure

Blood pressure, more precisely the mean arterial pressure (MAP), is a function of cardiac output and systemic vascular resistance (and the CVP, although its contribution is small and is therefore often omitted).

MAP = (CO x SVR) + CVP

In practical terms, a vasodilatory state with a low SVR, as seen in sepsis or systemic inflammation, will result in a low blood pressure, even with a normal or high cardiac output. A high SVR will lead to a high MAP provided the cardiac output is maintained and not reduced due to the increased afterload.

Systemic Vascular Resistance (SVR)

The systemic vascular resistance is often used to make a statement about the patient's circulatory state. In this context it is important to note that whilst the SVR can be *calculated* from the MAP, CVP and CO, it is not *determined* by them as seen above. Therefore, using the SVR as a marker of cardiovascular state is somewhat an oversimplification.

$$SVR = \frac{MAP - CVP}{CO}$$

From the SVR formula it becomes clear that both, a low MAP with normal CO or a normal MAP with a high cardiac output will result in a low *calculated* SVR. Conversely, a high MAP with normal CO or a normal MAP with a low cardiac output will result in a high *calculated* SVR.

The bottom line is that optimising the patient's cardiovascular status requires careful consideration of many factors including preload, afterload, contractility, oxygenation and peripheral resistance.

Normal and Abnormal Patient Progression

"Common things are common"

Certain physiological changes are expected following cardiac surgery. Of these, some may represent a predictable or expected departure of physiological variables from preoperative normal ranges, and others may be a sign of some significant or dangerous physiological derangement. It is important to recognise those changes that are significant or those that could be optimised through medical management. Most of these changes occur in the immediate postoperative phase and the patient's physiology usually returns to normal within a few days of the surgery.

Normal cardiovascular changes

Myocardial contractility reduces after cardiopulmonary bypass with cardioplegic arrest. While the surgeons aim to protect the myocardium as much as possible during the operation, it is simply impossible to achieve a normal level of cellular oxygenation. Although the heart has stopped beating, the myocardial cells still use energy and eventually deoxygenate and become progressively more acidotic. This leads to some reduced contractility in all hearts that are arrested for a period of time during the operation. Myocardial contractility is expected to reach its lowest point around 4 hours post bypass, and recovers over the next 1 to 3 days. This is why many units routinely monitor the cardiac output with a pulmonary artery catheter or have a low threshold for initiating cardiac output monitoring.

In addition, total body fluid also changes during cardiac surgery, and added intravenous fluid only temporarily increases intravascular volume. Ultimately, some of the fluid will leak out of the vessels due to increased capillary permeability, thereby causing peripheral oedema. Although fluid is given intra-operatively either as intravenous infusions or as pump prime and the total body fluid may increase by 20 – 30%, the patient may still be intravascularly depleted due to this capillary leakage and redistribution.

Normal respiratory changes

General anaesthesia, inhalational anaesthesia agents and cardiopulmonary bypass affect lung function. Atelectasis after cardiac surgery is common and contributes to ventilation-perfusion mismatch as well as reducing the functional capacity of the respiratory system which may already be compromised by pre-existing conditions such as COPD, asthma, recent chest infections, smoking or other pulmonary conditions. The respiratory system usually begins to return to its pre-operative state after 1-2 days. Gas exchange can be improved in the intubated patient by increasing the PEEP and FiO_2. However, respiratory mechanics are usually superior in a self-ventilating patient, if this can be achieved, and expeditious weaning from the ventilator and extubation are ideal for a good recovery.

Respiratory dynamics for the extubated patient can be improved by supplemental oxygen, adequate analgesia, minimisation of pulmonary oedema and early physiotherapy.

Normal renal response

The response of the kidneys is variable depending on various pre and peri-operative factors. In normal functioning kidneys with adequate renal reserve, excretion of the extra volume acquired during cardiopulmonary bypass results in several hours of polyuria. Serum urea and creatinine should not change significantly post-operatively in such cases.

A decrease in urine output can often be the very first sign of inadequate organ perfusion, caused by low cardiac output, low blood pressure or a combination of those two.

Gastro-intestinal System

Splanchnic blood flow, hepatic and pancreatic function are usually well maintained after CPB. However, due to capillary leakage, GI tract oedema may still occur and absorption of a number of substrates e.g. complex carbohydrates may be affected. Normally there is no major derangement in GI function post operatively.

Central Nervous System

Postoperative neurologic dysfunction occurs with considerable frequency post cardiac surgery, in large part due to the effect of micro-emboli. Risk factors for CNS dysfunction include:

- Advanced age
- Hypertension
- Diabetes mellitus
- Smoking
- Previous stroke
- Carotid stenosis
- Aortic atherosclerosis
- Poor left ventricular function
- Peripheral vascular disease
- Prolonged CPB or deep hypothermic circulatory arrest
- Peri-operative myocardial infarction
- Post-operative atrial fibrillation.

The incidence of a major cerebrovascular event is approximately 2% in the absence of other significant risk factors. More subtle neuro-psychometric changes such as agitation, confusion, mild depression and intellectual deficit are more common. These changes are typically transient during the early post-operative course and rapidly diminish with most patients making a full recovery.

Coagulopathy and bleeding

Cardiac surgery causes a postoperative bleeding tendency as a result of platelet dysfunction, thrombocytopenia, deficiencies in coagulation factors, inadequate heparin reversal, rebound anti-coagulation from excess protamine or fibrinolysis (blood contact with the biomaterial components of the heart-lung machine) and the occasional imperfect surgical haemostasis. Risks factors for significant bleeding include redo surgery, longer bypass times and bleeding increases with the complexity of the surgery. *There is no magic amount of bleeding which is normal!* It must be seen in context of the patient's pre and peri-operative states as well as the technique and criteria of the individual surgeon.

If a patient deviates from the expected post-operative course, it is important to work out why. Diagnosis in this setting often takes the form of recognising a pattern of problems. Most cases of non-progression are cardiac in origin, either due to primary pump failure or some secondary cause. Diagnosis should be early but should not delay emergency treatment pending investigations

The CALS Five-Point Plan (ADAIR)

Cardiac surgical patients can deteriorate rapidly. The response to this needs to be fast and well-coordinated. The organisation of such a response benefits from structure, which for the purposes of CALS is presented as the ADAIR five-point plan.

The acronym ADAIR stands for Assessment, Diagnosis, Action Plan, Investigations and Re-Assessment and is a toolkit for systematic, focused and effective management of a deteriorating cardiac surgical patient.

This structured approach to problems in the post-operative cardiac surgical patient facilitates prompt and accurate diagnosis and treatment as well as active communication.

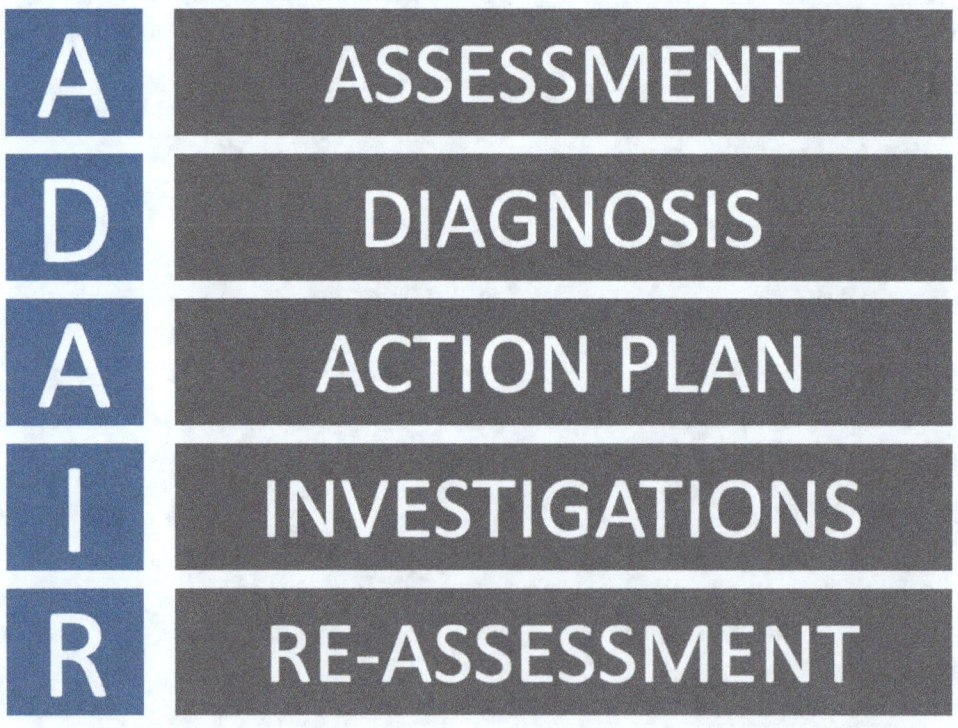

A – Assessment

The assessment is a rapid (2 minutes or less), focused examination of the patient. A more thorough clinical examination can be performed once the patient is stabilised. The objective of this initial assessment is to quickly identify major problems that require immediate treatment. It is analogous to the primary survey in the assessment of a trauma patient and follows a familiar DRSABCDE approach.

Danger

Wear personal protective equipment (PPE) (most importantly an apron, gloves and a face mask with eye shield) if there is any chance of exposure to body fluids. Patient aggression due to delirium or a pre-existing condition is also a risk to staff.

Response

Quickly assess the patient's conscious state. You can do a Glasgow Coma Score but it takes longer and is more complex compared to an AVPU score.

A – The patient is alert

V – The patient only responds to voice?

P – The patient only responds to a painful stimulus

U – The patient is unconscious

Send for help

A deteriorating cardiac surgical patient requires simultaneous assessment and management. The number of tasks will quickly multiply in the course of the initial assessment. It is therefore essential to access additional nursing and medical staff in the early stages of assessment, anticipating an increase in the complexity of the situation, instead of waiting for further patient deterioration. Senior medical and surgical staff (eg. the intensivist and cardiac surgeon) should be contacted at the earliest opportunity.

Airway

If the patient is speaking with a normal voice and no added noises, the airway is patent. Signs suggestive of a threatened airway include stridor, loud wheeze, coughing, or an abnormal seesaw movement of the chest.

If the patient is unconscious and not intubated, open and check the airway with a head tilt, chin lift and jaw thrust. Suction any secretions.

If the patient is intubated, check endotracheal tube (ETT) patency with a suction catheter and check endotracheal position with end-tidal CO_2. Disconnect from the ventilator and bag ventilate with 100% oxygen to get a feeling for airway resistance. If the ETT is in the correct position and patent, you may put the patient back on the ventilator.

Breathing

Respiratory assessment can be completed rapidly using the "look, listen and feel" approach familiar from the ALS and EMST protocols. Look for bilaterally equal chest movement, auscultate for breath sounds, and feel the patients' chest to assess chest expansion.

Auscultate both sides of the lungs, apices and bases, looking for crepitations, wheeze or absent breath sounds. Hypoxia needs to be addressed immediately by increasing the FiO_2 to 100%, even for patients thought to be "CO2 retainers".

Exclude a pneumothorax or haemothorax by percussion, an urgent x-ray and lung ultrasound.

Circulation

Assess the peripheral circulation by feeling the temperature of the patients' extremities. Whether the patient's hands and feet feel warm, or cold and clammy, could help discriminate between different shock states.

Check heart rate and rhythm including pacemaker function. When assessing the blood pressure, take into account whether the patient is on vasopressors, inotropes or other vasoactive drugs.

If available, check invasive pressures and measure a cardiac output. Look for pulse pressure variation in the arterial pressure waveform ("swing") where the amplitude varies with respiration, which may indicate hypovolaemia and/or fluid responsiveness. A bedside ultrasound will also be helpful to determine volume status and cardiac contractility.

Though urine output may not be perfectly accurate as a measure of organ perfusion in the immediate postoperative state, it should be noted as a part of the circulatory assessment.

Chest drain output is another essential part of the circulatory system assessment. Check the tubing as well as the drain bottle. Though there may not be any specific "normal" drain output value, specific red flags include a sudden increase, or decrease, in the drain output. A constant flow which has suddenly stopped may indicate that the drain has become blocked.

Disability

After the ABC assessment has excluded immediate threats to the patient's life, there should now be enough time to perform a more detailed neurological exam, focusing on GCS, pupils, and focal lateralising signs.

If the patient is alert, check whether they are oriented to person, time and place. Confusion is often the first sign of sepsis or of a stroke. "D" is also a reminder to check the BSL.

Exposure

The initial assessment needs to include a thorough examination of the patient's skin, lines and wounds. Expose the patient and examine them from head to toe. Look for any rashes, redness, discharge or ecchymosis. Bleeding from venous harvest sites is a common cause of haemodynamic instability which could be missed without thorough exposure and examination.

Check the lines and wounds for any redness or discharge.

D - Diagnosis

The information produced in the course of the structured DRSABCDE assessment should be enough to guide a provisional diagnosis for the cause of the patient's deterioration. If not, there should be enough information to at least make a "best guess" and treat the immediately life threatening physiological abnormalities.

By far the most common complication in the early postoperative phase is hypotension. There are only a handful of common causes: y hypovolaemia, low cardiac output, vasoplegia and arrhythmias. These are discussed in detail in chapter 4.

A – Action Plan

Armed with a provisional diagnosis, it should now be possible to formulate an action plan and communicate it to the team. Effective communication and allocation of tasks is important to ensure successful team management (see Chapter 6, Human Factors). To discuss the provisional diagnosis and management with the team has the added benefit of sharing a mental model of the situation, allowing team members to offer their own insights and to be able to predict the next necessary steps in the management.

Of note, the Action Plan comes before Investigations. Often there is not enough time to wait for results of investigations to come back. In those circumstances, the patient must be stabilised first.

I - Investigations

Given the rapidly changing dynamic patient condition and the timeframe of the deterioration, the number of possible investigations available at this stage may be limited.

The following rapidly available investigations may help to confirm or refute the provisional diagnosis:

- ABG/VBG to check Hb, lactate and electrolytes
- FBC, coagulation profile, fibrinogen, ACT, TEG or ROTEM to determine whether the patient needs blood- or clotting products
- Echocardiography (transoesophageal as required) and lung ultrasound to assess cardiac function and to look for pericardial tamponade and pleural collections

- Chest radiograph to look for pulmonary and pleural pathologies

R – Re-Assess

Following the implementation of a management plan, the patient needs to be reassessed to determine their response, and to guide any adjustments to the management strategy. Many interventions can produce undesirable adverse effects and these need to be identified before they develop into major complications (for example, fluid overload from aggressive resuscitation, or haemorrhage from a newly inserted chest drain).

Hypotension

Hypotension is the most common post-operative cardiac surgical emergency. Prompt treatment can keep the patient alive awaiting help and results. Causes may be multifactorial; constant reassessment of one cause of hypotension may uncover another, thus, reassessment is mandatory.

A simple approach to hypotension is to consider the blood pressure as requiring 3 main factors:

·   **Preload (adequate volume)**

·   **Afterload (vascular resistance)**

·   **Contractility**

Additionally, rate (adequate cardiac output, enough time for diastolic filling) and rhythm (atrial kick, ventricular synchrony) are important for blood pressure.

After establishing whether the problem is with preload, afterload or contractility, one can refine one's diagnosis with further investigation. Although there may be an issue with one of these factors, any given patient may have a combination of several concurrent problems. No single sign or measurement is reliable on its own, and a "multimodal" assessment is always required. Fortunately, the post-op cardiac surgical patient is usually well monitored, offering several methods of rapidly assessing their cardiovascular performance:

·   A quick focused history, aiming to assess risk factors in the patient's background medical history and perioperative course

·   Clinical examination, focusing on peripheral perfusion

·   Assessment of arterial line "swing" or pulse pressure variation

·   Assessment of the CVP or JVP

·   Assessment of cardiac output monitoring device measurements

Low preload as the cause of hypotension

Hypovolemia is the most common cause of post-operative hypotension.

Factors which might make you think that preload is the problem include:

·   **History**

    -    Recent return from theatre (i.e. first 0-6 hours)

    -    Pre-operative use of antiplatelet agents

    -    Emergency surgery (vs. elective)

- Large drain output

- Recent vigorous diuresis

· **Clinical findings**

- Dry mucous membranes

- Poor skin turgor

- Tachycardia

- Signs of bleeding

- Poor capillary refill

· **Measurements**

- A low CVP.
  A high CVP does not exclude a preload problem, but a low CVP in a hypotensive patient strongly suggests that the patient may be underfilled

- A low diastolic pressure

- A low pulmonary artery diastolic pressure

- A low pulmonary artery wedge pressure (PAWP)

- A high SVRI measurement (above 2400 dynes · $sec/cm^5/m^2$)

- A low cardiac index or cardiac output measurement

· **Dynamic features**

- Pulse pressure variation, otherwise known as a "swing" in the arterial line

- A vigorous blood pressure response to small amounts of fluid resuscitation

The most important cause of hypovolaemia following cardiac surgery is blood loss. Drain output is an essential part of examining these patients (though blood loss from other sites, e.g. the pleura, vein harvest site or retroperitoneum, is also possible).

- A small fluid bolus (250-500ml) is a good immediate strategy for hypovolaemic patients as it is unlikely to cause harm.

- At the same time, a blood gas should be processed, looking for a drop in haemoglobin. Remember that haemoglobin takes a few minutes to fall following an acute haemorrhage and blood transfusion should be administered regardless in this circumstance.

- Coagulopathy should be assessed concurrently. Platelet count, APTT, PT and fibrinogen should be tested. Point-of-care testing such as TEG or ROTEM may yield a faster result than laboratory coagulation studies. Again, in acute haemorrhage, factor transfusion should not be withheld in the presence of normal laboratory values as these take time to derange.

- It is important to note that early cardiac tamponade, which is also transiently fluid-responsive, may mimic the findings of hypovolaemia, and that the two conditions often coexist in this setting.

Cardiac tamponade as the cause of hypotension

Cardiac tamponade is the most rapidly progressive and dangerous cause of post-operative hypotension, and should be one of the first differential diagnoses

- **History**
  - Recent return from theatre (i.e. first 0-6 hours)
  - High drain output; OR: minimal/zero drain output
  - Predisposition to bleeding (eg. pre-operative use of antiplatelet agents, emergency surgery, coagulopathy, acidosis)

- **Clinical findings**
  - Engorged neck veins
  - Cool extremities
  - Faint pulse, or pulsus paradoxus (where the pulse disappears entirely during a part of the respiratory cycle)
  - Sluggish capillary refill

- **Measurements**
  - A high CVP. Usually this is a progressive increase in CVP, to over 20 or even 30 mmHg.
  - A high SVRI measurement (above 2390 dynes · sec/cm^5/m^2)
  - A low cardiac index or cardiac output measurement
  - Electrical alternans
  - TTE or TOE evidence of cardiac tamponade

- **Dynamic features**
  - Pulse pressure variation, otherwise known as a "swing" in the arterial line.
  - Blood pressure response is transient (i.e. hypotension develops again, as soon as the fluid bolus has finished)

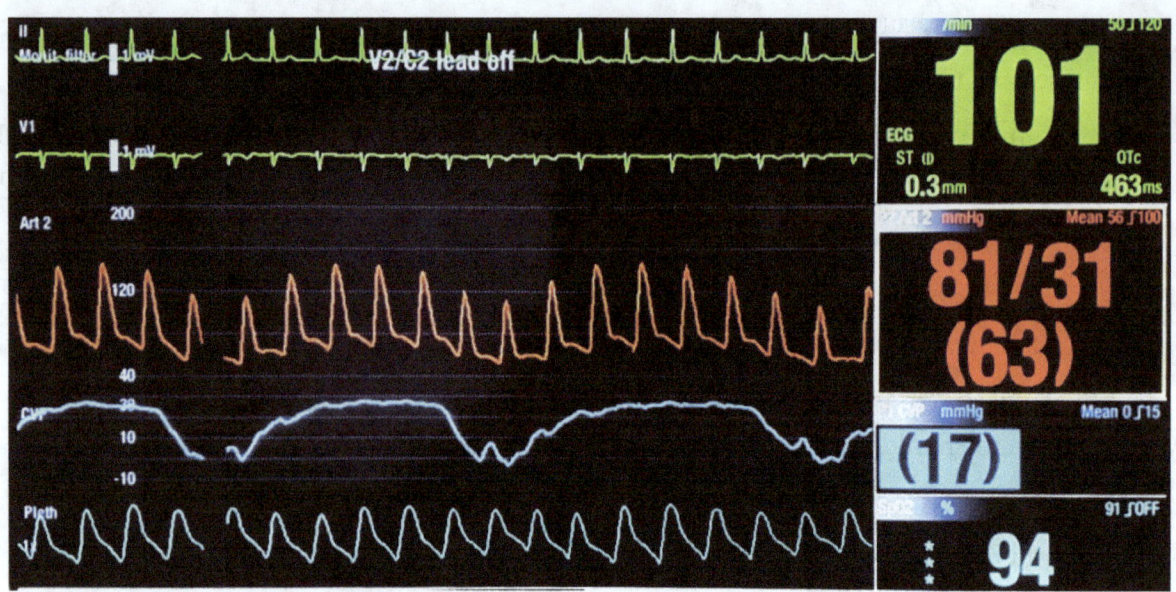

A typical monitor appearance of a patient with cardiac tamponade. There is tachycardia and hypotension, with a high CVP (mean of 17, but rising up to 30 during the respiratory cycle), and a very obvious arterial pulse pressure variation ("swing").

Cardiac tamponade is usually a surgical emergency. A multidisciplinary approach to management is required

- Alert the surgical and anaesthesia team. Often the patient will need transoesophageal echocardiography and return to surgery.

- Administer a fluid bolus (250-500ml) – this may be a way to maintain organ perfusion while waiting for definitive therapy

- Assess for bleeding and coagulopathy. Remember that cardiac tamponade and haemorrhage can coexist.

Low afterload (vasoplegia) as the cause of hypotension

"Vasoplegia", or poor peripheral vascular resistance, is a common cause of postoperative hypotension. Factors that suggest vascular resistance is the culprit include

· **History**

- Prolonged operating time or cardiopulmonary bypass time
- Pre-operative infection
- Pre-operative use of antihypertensives (esp. ACE-inhibitors)

· **Clinical findings**

- Warm extremities
- Brisk capillary refill
- Widened pulse pressure, which manifests as a bounding pulse

- A hyperdynamic praecordium

- A raised temperature

· **Measurements**

- A low diastolic pressure

- A low SVRI measurement (below 2000 dynes · sec/cm^5/m^2)

- A normal cardiac index or cardiac output measurement

· **Dynamic features**

- An absence of clear pulse pressure variation, or "swing" in the arterial line

- The lack of a vigorous response to a fluid bolus

Decreased peripheral vascular resistance responds to vasopressors. Noradrenaline is the vasopressor of choice for post-operative cardiac surgical patients who have central vascular access. Peripheral metaraminol (as intermittent boluses or infusion) is a valid alternative.

Beware of hypotension that is labelled as 'vasoplegia' which fails to respond to vasopressors. If the vasopressor dose has increased significantly without much impact on the blood pressure, there is probably another problem – most likely with contractility.

Poor contractility as the cause of hypotension

Poor cardiac contractility is another common cause of postoperative hypotension. Factors that suggest that poor contractility is at fault for the low blood pressure include

· **History**

- Prolonged operating time or cardiopulmonary bypass time

- Pre-existing poor LV function

- Emergency surgery for an acute problem (eg. following a recent STEMI)

· **Clinical findings**

- Cool extremities

- Sluggish or absent capillary refill, mottling

- Narrow pulse pressure and a thready faint pulse

· **Measurements**

- A high CVP

- A very high SVRI measurement (well above 2400 dynes · sec/cm^5/m^2)

- A low cardiac index or cardiac output measurement

- A high pulmonary artery wedge pressure (PAWP)

· **Dynamic features**

- An absence of pulse pressure variation or "swing"

- Nil or minimal response to a fluid bolus

- Unexpected lack of response to vasopressor infusion titration

Poor cardiac contractility requires inotropes. The choice of inotrope depends on the cardiac physiology and is individualised to each patient. Broadly speaking:

- **Adrenaline** is a reliable positive inotrope with vasopressor effects. One of the disadvantages is the tendency to produce hyperlactatemia, which degrades the utility of lactate in the assessment of the shocked patient

- **Dobutamine** is an inotrope often chosen to support poor contractility where poor left ventricular function is the main problem

- **Milrinone** is an inodilator which can improve cardiac performance where right heart function is more impaired than left, as it can act as a pulmonary vasodilator and decrease RV afterload

- **Levosimendan** is an inodilator with a different mechanism of action and longer duration of action, which can also improve RV afterload.

Beware that positive inotropes increase cardiac contractility at the expense of increased myocardial oxygen consumption and increased risk of arrhythmia. Inotrope therapy should be combined with a vigilant correction of abnormal electrolytes, particularly of potassium and magnesium. Additionally, "inodilator" agents such as milrinone and levosimendan may cause a decrease in peripheral vascular resistance and produce worsening hypotension.

In patients who have an inadequate response to inotropes, mechanical haemodynamic support may be required, such as intra-aortic balloon counterpulsation or ECMO.

Quick reference table

	Extremities	Pulse	Pulse pressure variation (arterial line "swing")	CVP
Hypovolemia	Cool extremities	Faint	Present	Low
Vasoplegia	Warm extremities	Bounding	Absent	Variable
Low contractility	Cool extremities	Faint	Absent	High
Tamponade	Cool extremities	Faint	Very obvious	Very high

Arrhythmia and tachycardia as the cause of hypotension

Patients recovering from cardiac surgery frequently develop rhythm and rate disturbances which result in hypotension. These include:

·   **Bradycardia or heart block,** which requires pacing or positive chronotrope agents such as isoprenaline (isoproterenol)

·   **Atrial tachyarrhythmia,** such as AF, flutter or SVT, which may require antiarrhythmic agents or synchronised direct current cardioversion

Sinus tachycardia is usually the *result* of hypotension, rather than its cause. A sinus tachycardia should be regarded as a compensation for hypotension, and causes of hypotension should be investigated.

Pacing

Indications for pacing

Post-operative patients commonly have epicardial pacing wires which should be connected to a pacemaker. Pacing can also be achieved transcutaneously in an emergency. Predominant rhythms amenable to pacing are asystole, complete heart block and severe bradycardia.

Pacemaker terminology

- **Sensitivity** of a pacemaker electrode is the minimum myocardial voltage required to be detected as a P wave or R wave, measured in mV.

- **Output** of a pacemaker is the current (in mA) which it produces as a brief pulse.

- **Capture** is the effective stimulation of cardiac depolarisation by the pacemaker.

- **Mechanical capture** is the association of a paced ECG QRS with an arterial pulse.

- **Capture threshold** is the minimum amount of current (in mA) required to initiate depolarization of the paced chamber.

- **Output failure** is the failure to produce a pacing spike.

- **Failure to capture** is where the pacing spikes do not produce QRS complexes.

- **Undersensing** is where the pacemaker paces asynchronously in spite of the presence of obvious P or QRS waves.

- **Oversensing** is the failure to pace in spite of bradycardia, when electrical signals are inappropriately recognised as native cardiac activity and pacing is inhibited.

Pacemaker mode nomenclature

- Pacemaker modes are described by the NBG (a combination of American and British society terms) pacemaker code, which consists of five letters; in the cardiac surgical post-op setting, only the first three letters are in routine use.

Chambers paced	Chambers Sensed	Mode of response (what the pacemaker will do if activity in the sensed chamber is detected)
V = ventricle	V = ventricle	T = triggered
A = atrium	A = atrium	I = inhibited
D = dual (A and V)	D = dual (A and V)	D = dual (triggered or inhibited)
O = none	O = none	O = none

Thus, a pacemaker in a VOO mode paces the ventricle completely asynchronously; a pacemaker in AAI mode paces the atrium and is inhibited by spontaneous atrial activity, and a DDD pacemaker will pace either chamber on demand (i.e. if the spontaneous rate is inadequate, or if the atrial electrical activity fails to activate the ventricle).

Normal settings for temporary ventricular epicardial pacing wires:

- **Output:** **10 mA**
- **Sensitivity:** **2 mV**
- **Rate:** **80**

Routine care for epicardial pacing wires

- Sensitivity and capture thresholds should be checked at least daily.
- When no longer in use, the wires need to be wrapped in gauze and attached to the patient's chest with dressings.
- Usually, wires are removed on day 4 or 5 post op.
- If the patient is anticoagulated, the INR should ideally be below 1.5 in order for the removal to be safe.

Checking pacemaker threshold

- Set the pacemaker rate 10-20 beats above the native rate.
- Start reducing the output until a QRS complex no longer follows each pacing spike.
- The output at which capture is lost is the capture threshold.
- Typically, one might want to set the output to about double this capture threshold.

Checking pacemaker sensitivity

- The patient must have a native rhythm.
- Put the pacemaker in a VVI, AAI or DDD mode.
- Set the output as low as possible (you only need to see the pacing spikes).
- Change the rate to one which is 10-20 beats lower than the patient's native rate (sense indicator should be flashing).
- Raise the sensitivity value until no cardiac activity is sensed (pace indicator is flashing).
- Now, keep lowering the sensitivity value until the pacemaker senses every p-wave or QRS interval (sense indicator is flashing again).
- This minimal sensitivity value is the sensitivity threshold.
- Leave the sensitivity turned down to half of the sensitivity threshold.

Pacemaker operation during a cardiac arrest

- **VF:** the pacemaker should be turned off.
- **Asystole:** the pacemaker should be set to VOO mode, to pace asynchronously.
- **PEA with pacing spikes:** the pacemaker should be turned off, as pacing spikes and paced waves can mask ventricular fibrillation.

Pacemaker rhythm interpretation

Normal AAI mode

Pacing spikes appear before the P-wave, QRS is normal (narrow).

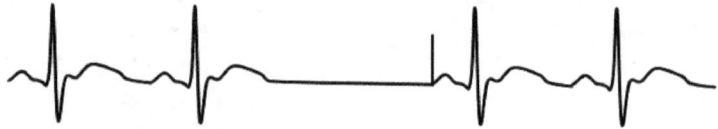

In the presence of normal atrial activity, the pacemaker does not pace.

Normal VVI mode

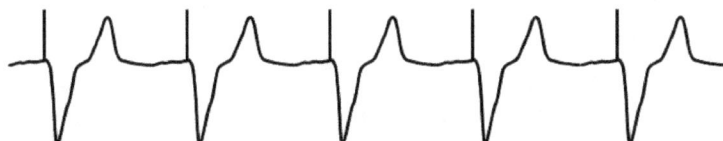

Pacing spikes appear before the QRS complex, QRS is wide (LBBB morphology).

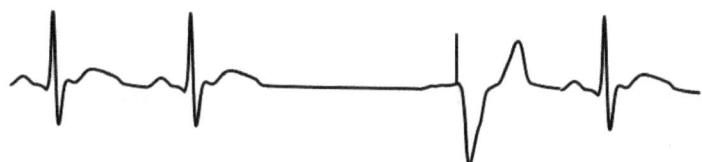

In the presence of normal sinus rhythm, the pacemaker does not pace.

Normal DDD mode

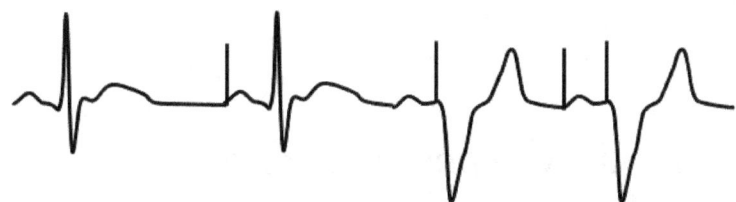

In the presence of normal sinus rhythm, the pacemaker does not pace. If atrial activity is absent, the pacemaker paces the atrium. If atrial activity does not produce a ventricular depolarisation (eg. AV node block), the pacemaker paces the ventricle, and the resulting QRS is broad. If neither chamber is active, the pacemaker paces both chambers.

Common abnormal pacemaker rhythms

Output failure

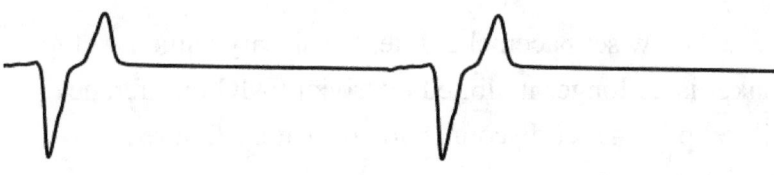

No pacing spikes. Pacemaker may be disconnected or out of battery power ("oversensing" is also possible).

Failure to capture

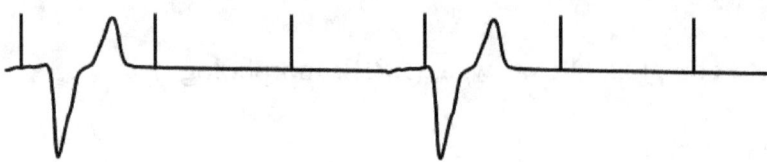

Pacing spikes occur at regular intervals, but they are not followed by consistent QRS complexes or P waves. Increase the output.

Failure to sense ("undersensing")

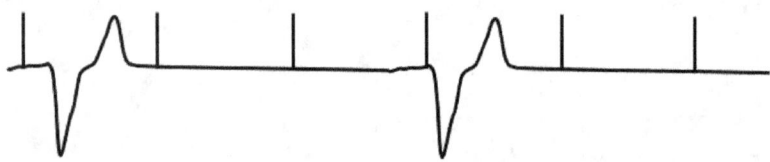

Observed in any inhibited sensing mode (AAI, VVI or DDD). Native rhythm is adequate, but the pacemaker is still pacing at the set rate.
This could cause VT/VF due to R-on-T phenomenon.
Sensitivity value is set too high: check sensitivity threshold and then set pacemaker to half of that value.

"Oversensing"

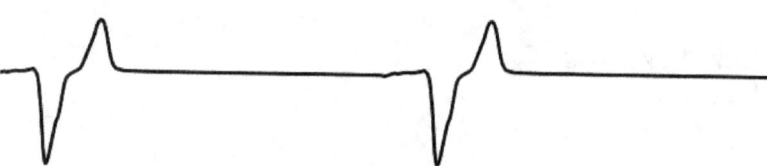

No pacing spikes in spite of native rate below set pacemaker rate. Sensitivity value is set too low; increase the value until pacemaker is no longer inhibited by trivial EMG interference (this could also represent output failure: pacemaker disconnection or battery failure is an alternative explanation for this lack of pacing spikes).

Human factors

Necessary staff: the 6 key roles

The CALS-ANZ protocol defines clear role allocations and each of those roles should be taken by an appropriately trained team member. Individual roles and teamwork should be regularly practised in interprofessional and interdisciplinary simulation training (CALS-ANZ 10.2). The 6 key roles are:

1. Team leader

2. ICU coordinator

3. Resternotomy team (generally 2 staff members)

4. Resternotomy trolley

5. Defibrillator and pacing

6. Airway and breathing

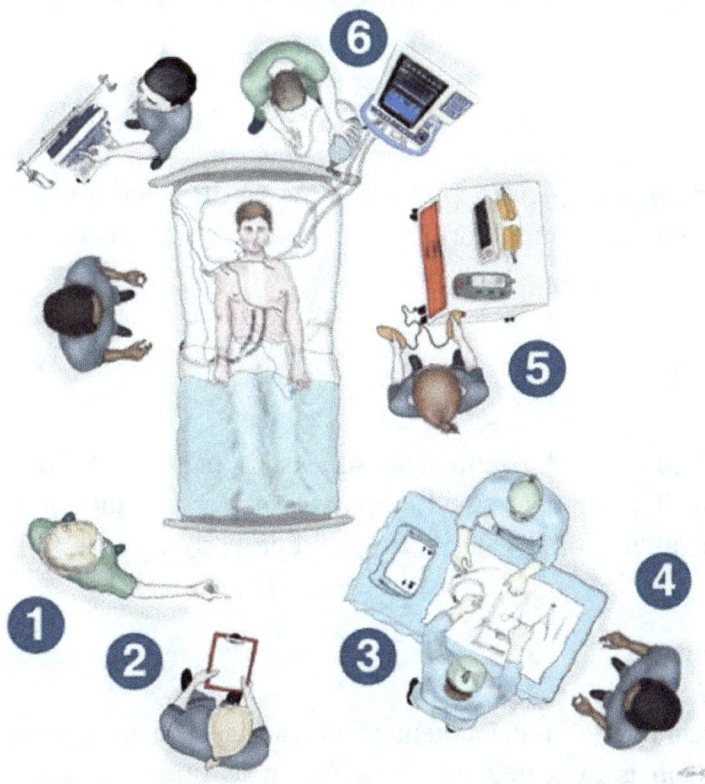

Six key roles for staff managing a CALS emergency have been identified through experience and simulation:

- Chest compressions
- Airway
- Defibrillation
- Team leader
- Drugs
- Coordinator

Additionally, a resternotomy team (ideally consisting of two people) is required.

Chest compressions

Once the cardiac arrest has been established, one person is allocated to perform chest compressions. This should commence at a rate of 100-120 beats per minute while looking at the arterial trace to assess effectiveness. The only exception to this is when immediate defibrillation or pacing is appropriate prior to the commencement of chest compressions.

Airway and breathing

The 2nd rescuer increases the inspired oxygen to 100%, removes PEEP, and assesses airway and breathing specifically to exclude pneumothorax, haemothorax or an endotracheal tube problem.

Defibrillation

This person connects the defibrillator and administers shocks, if indicated. They are also assigned to manage pacing, and if emergency resternotomy is performed they must ensure that the internal defibrillator is available on the sterile field and properly connected.

Team leader

This senior person should conduct overall management of the cardiac arrest, ensuring that the protocol is followed and a person is allocated to each role. In addition the senior person ensures a team quickly prepares for resternotomy.

Drug administration

This person stops all infusions once initial resuscitative efforts have failed, administers amiodarone and manages other drugs or infusions as appropriate.

Coordinator

This role, typically a charge nurse or senior nursing unit leader, coordinates activity peripheral to the bedside. This includes preparing for potential resternotomy as soon as a cardiac arrest is called, directing available personnel and calling for expert assistance if not immediately available while continually reporting progress to the team leader.

Resternotomy team

In addition to the six key roles above, a resternotomy team should be identified and immediately gown and glove preparing for emergency resternotomy. This should occur **immediately upon identifying a cardiac arrest**, rather than waiting until other conservative attempts at resuscitation have failed. Due to the fact that arrest due to tamponade is always a possibility, this team must be sufficiently trained to always be able to perform a resternotomy within 5 minutes of arrest in the intensive care unit.

Preemptive role allocation

It is good practice to allocate staff at every shift to make sure that, in the event of an emergency, there is a group of pre-allocated staff who each know their role. This is a practice which is becoming widespread in busy cardiothoracic intensive care units. The discussion should take place at the beginning of each medical and nursing shift. Key staff can be identified with stickers, lanyards, or any other suitable methods. The objective of this is to remove the need for cognitive processing of role allocation in the emergency event, so as to free the team leader to focus on the clinical problem.

Crowd control

A cardiac arrest emergency announcement in a large ICU can bring a large crowd who increase the chaos of the situation without necessarily bringing anything beneficial. Apart from adding noise and distraction, these staff can get in the way of the scrubbed resternotomy team, or obstruct access for staff bringing essential equipment. It is often necessary to actively dismiss these extra staff. This possible seventh role can be allocated to a senior nurse or medical staff member, or the ICU coordinator can be asked to perform this role.

Shared mental model

It helps to have the CALS algorithm printed and available in every CTICU room. The CALS algorithm should also be a prominent feature of regular simulation and multidisciplinary team training. Familiarity with the algorithm and regular exposure to simulated CALS events is an essential part of forming a "shared mental model", i.e. the same basic understanding of the necessary steps shared by all team members.

Direct instructions and closed loop communication

To ensure that the team leader's instructions are followed, the directions being issued should be to the specific team member, rather than to the team as a whole. For example, instead asking "Can somebody call the surgeons?" it is better to directly instruct: "Tom, can you please call the surgical consultant". The team member executing the order should then complete the loop by responding to the team leader when the task has been completed, eg. "I've called the surgeon and they are on their way".

Graded assertiveness

No single team member should ever be afraid to point out a risk, a concern, or an actual or potential error. A graded approach is recommended to communicate this concern, escalating in urgency in proportion to the urgency of the situation, or if the concern is dismissed:

- **Curiosity/check:** "I wonder whether we should prepare for a resternotomy?"

- **Concern/option:** "I am concerned we're not getting much output. I think we should open the chest"

- **Crisis/emergency demand:** "We must open the chest now"

Equipment

It is important to recognise that emergency resternotomy is not a completely sterile procedure. There is usually not enough time for a thorough scrub hand wash, and therefore alcohol or chlorhexidine based hand rubs are suggested prior to donning sterile gloves and a sterile gown. Care should be taken to maintain sterility for the procedure field and equipment trolley. An all-in-one sterile drape is useful for the procedure field.

One reason for delay in emergency resternotomy is the preparation of a full sternotomy instrument set which may contain over 30 items of equipment, although only 5 items are essential: a scalpel, a wire cutter, a heavy needle holder, a single piece sternal retractor and a sucker (Figure 1). Larger sets are unnecessary in the setting of an emergency resternotomy and may confuse staff unaccustomed to assisting in surgery. In addition, when the operating team arrives, the full instrument set may be lost or contaminated when opened emergently by the ICU staff.

CALS-ANZ recommends that every unit is equipped with an emergency resternotomy set containing contents that every staff member is familiar with. This set should contain at least the minimum 5 items and back-up sets should be available. A full sternotomy set from theatres can be opened after the initial resternotomy is performed.

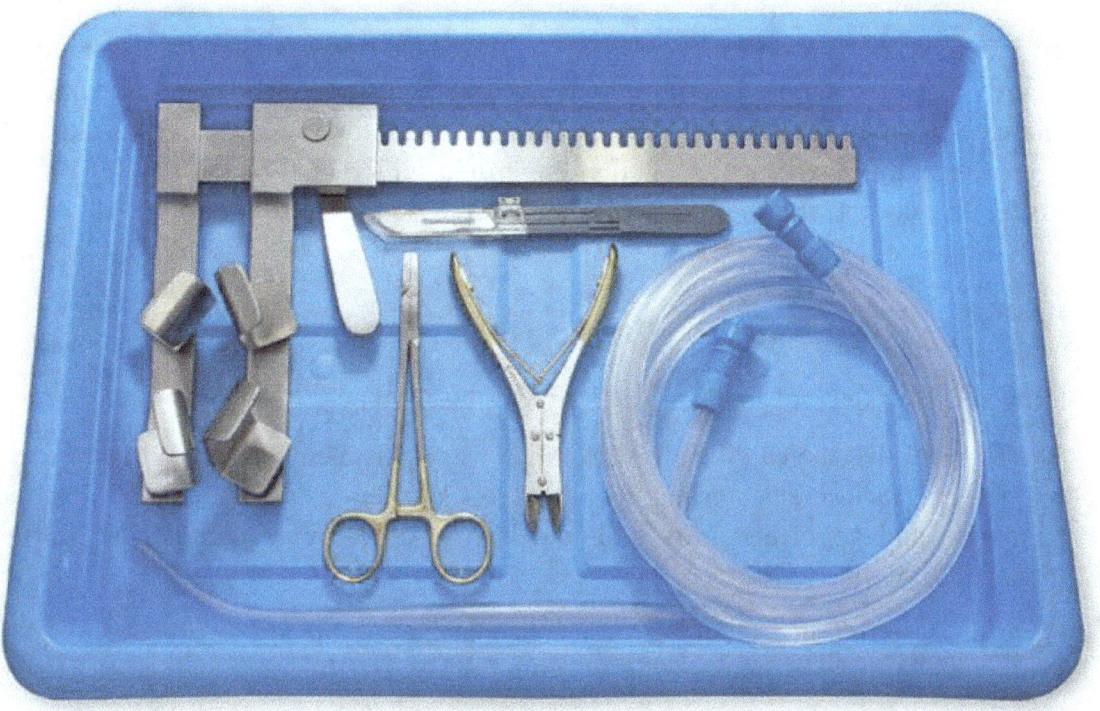

Figure 1. Above: The 5 essential items.

Once donned, the internal defibrillation paddles can be connected to the defibrillator with the correct positioning for internal defibrillation paddles.

Surgery for CALS

Opening the chest

Emergency resternotomy is a skill that many on a critical care unit involved in the treatment of post-operative cardiac surgical patients will need to learn. But whilst the resternotomy itself is relatively simple to perform, the rationale for what to do afterwards to aid in the resuscitation of the patient who has arrested after cardiac surgery can be seemingly complex. Despite this relative complexity the 'principles' of what to do are straightforward.

Resternotomy

Resternotomy should take place in a simple circumscribed manner.

1)   The moment that the cardiac arrest is called, two staff members should immediately put on PPE (face shield, sterile gown and gloves). There is no role for a full surgical handwash and gown and gloves should be put on as rapidly and in as sterile a manner as possible.

2)   Once the resternotomy team has indicated that they are ready to proceed, the team leader should instruct the person performing the external cardiac massage (ECM) to stop and to take off the dressing over the sternotomy wound as they step aside.

3)   The resternotomy team now deploys the one piece drape. Instructions for the use of such drapes can be seen at many online resources and in this handbook. Ideally, the drape covers the entire bed area to allow for sterile placement of the resternotomy set and the internal defibrillator paddles.

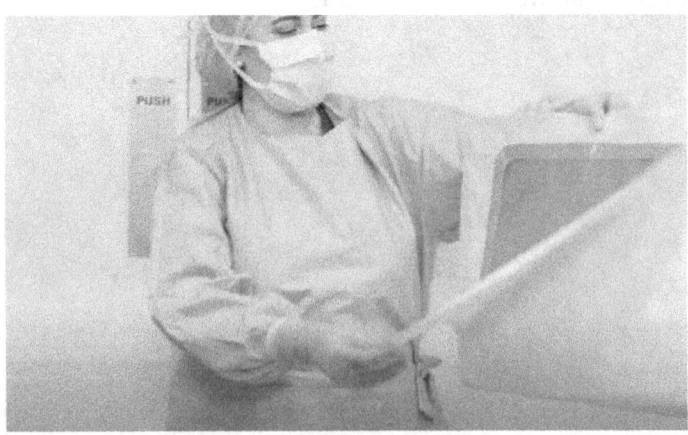

The drape is opened in a sterile manner

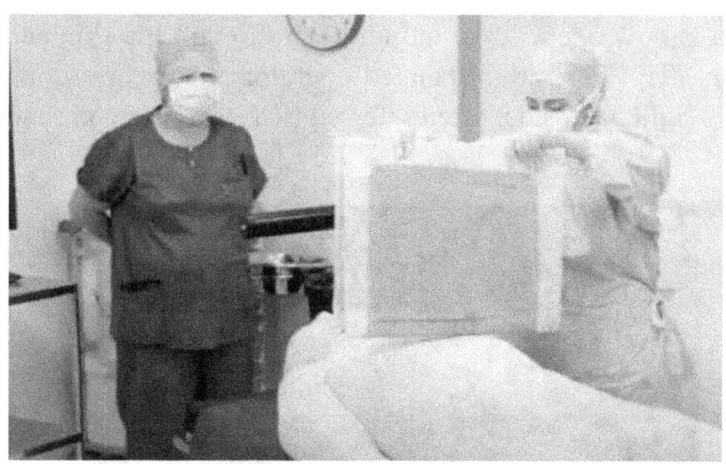

It is placed onto the patient

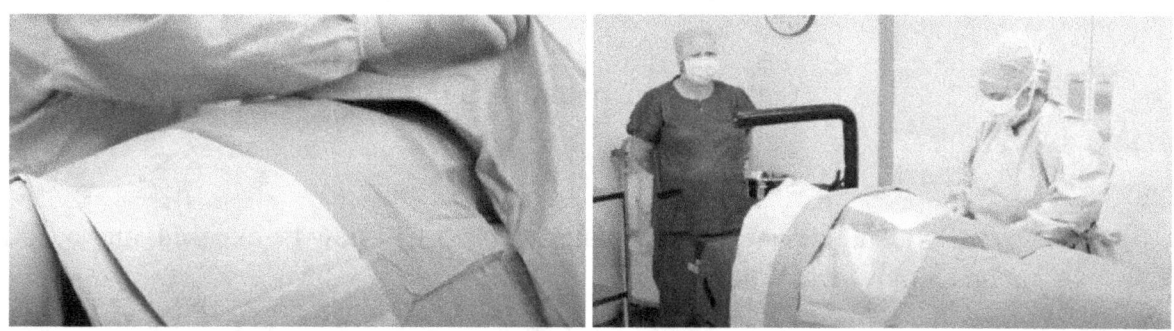

The distal part of the drape is opened over the feet

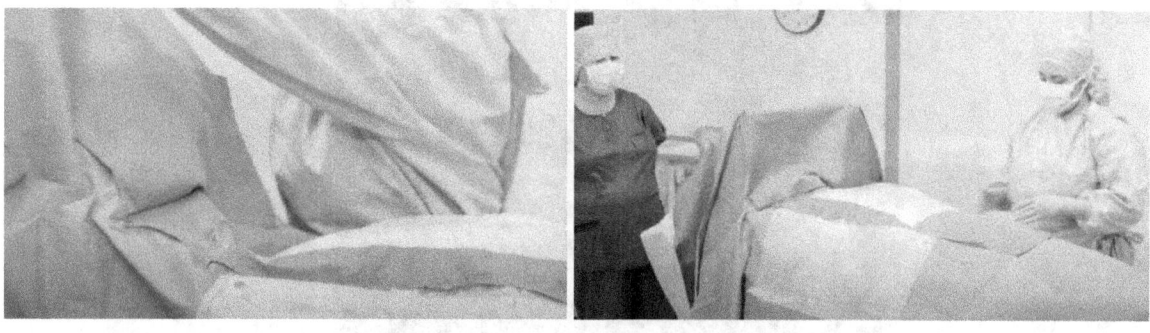

The proximal part is opened over the head

4) Once the drape has been positioned, one person recommences ECM whilst the other one is handed the resternotomy set and the internal defibrillator paddles in a sterile manner. The assistant now arranges them as appropriate in a sterile manner on the drape to allow for easy access. The connector of the defibrillator paddles is handed to the staff member assigned to operate the defibrillator. Finally, the suction is prepared by connecting the Yankauer tip to the tubing, which is handed out to an assistant for connection to the wall suction. .

5)   The wound is now opened by cutting down through the skin sutures, directly onto the sternum. (Tip: For a right-handed operator, this is best done when standing on the patient's right hand side, often referred to as the 'surgeon's side')

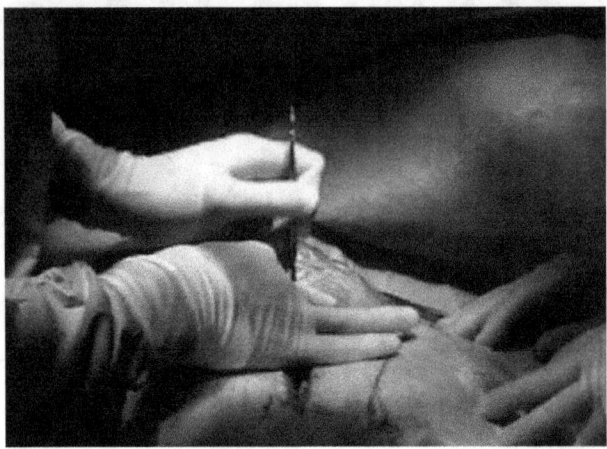

'Cutting down' onto the sternum

6)   The sternal closure devices (wires, plates, cables) will now be exposed, and need to be cut and removed.

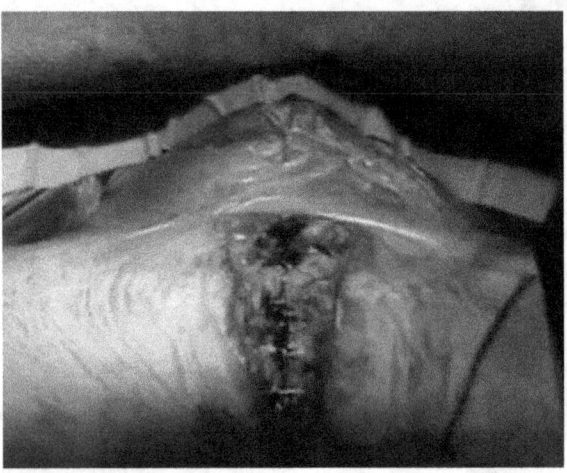

Sternal wires exposed after incision down to sternum

For wires, the cut should be just adjacent to the knot in the sternal wire whilst the wire is pulled upwards on the knot itself. All wires pulled out should be put into a sterile receiver and counted at the end of the procedure to ensure none have been lost.

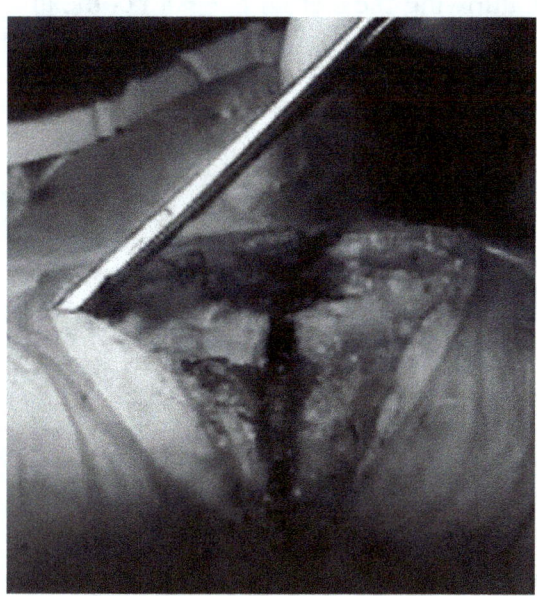

Removing sternal wires

For sternal plates, only the 'bridges' of the plates are cut in the middle whilst the two, now separated halves of the plates remain attached to the sternum.

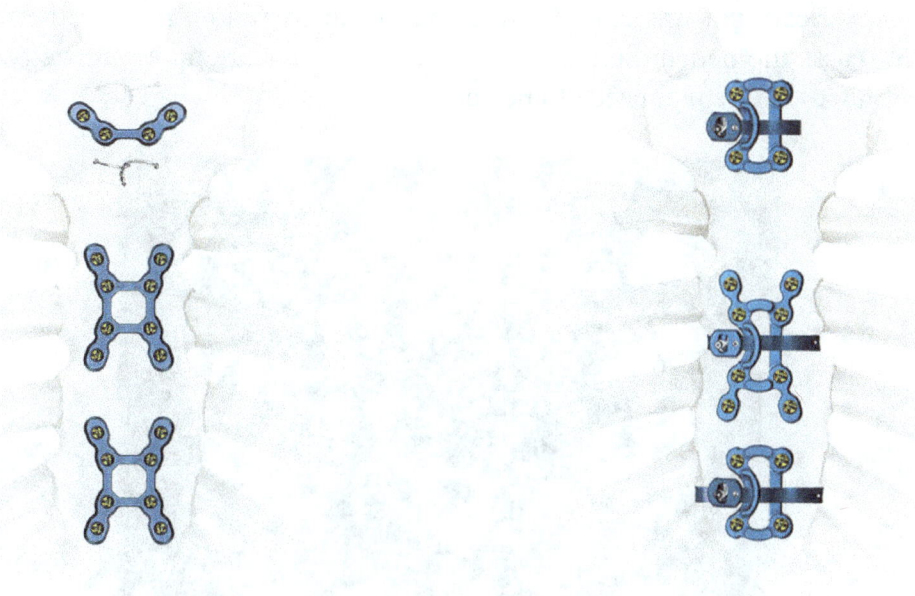

Note that occasionally a combination of different closing devices are used. The type of closure device used should be communicated to the critical care team.

7)   If the patient has a pericardial tamponade the very act of removing the sternal closure devices and allowing the sternal edges to come apart may well relieve it and allow for the return of an adequate cardiac output. (If this is the case, it is appropriate to wait for an experienced surgical team to arrive)

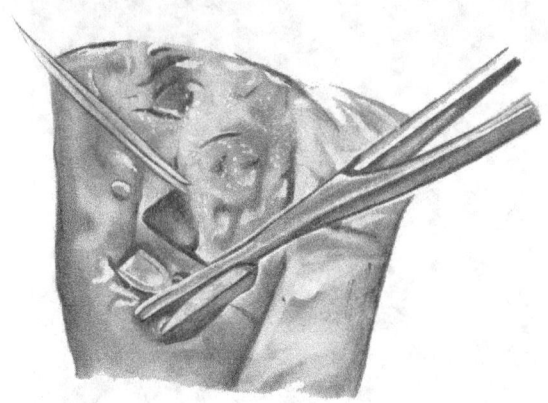

Sternum - open with all wires out

8)   The Sternal retractor should now be placed with care and the chest opened wide enough to expose the heart and to allow enough space between the retractor arms for bimanual internal cardiac massage. Adequate exposure also allows for the visualisation of any large active bleeding points and stops any clot tamponading the heart and reducing cardiac output

9)   If the pericardium was closed at the end of the operation, it has to be re-opened. In most cases the pericardium and extrapleural tissues are approximated with a single continuous suture that needs to be cut.

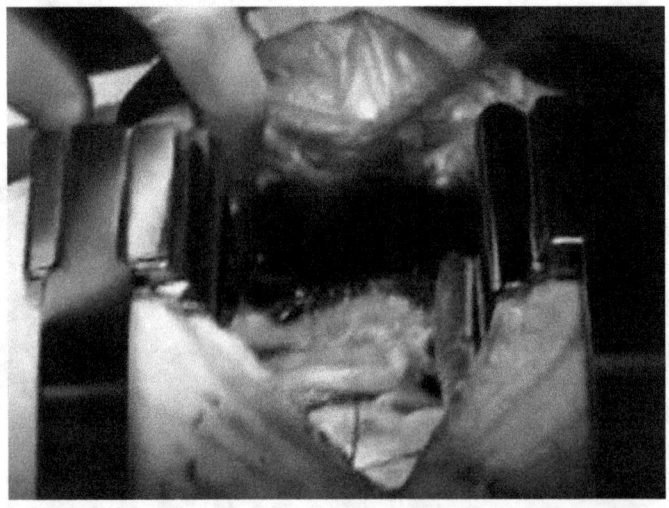

Sternal retractor in - note the chest drain in view

10) The end of the drains in the chest should now be pulled out of the way and tucked under the 'bridge' of the retractor to allow for maximum visibility of the heart.

11) Any blood clot overlying the heart should now be carefully removed using the Yankauer sucker.

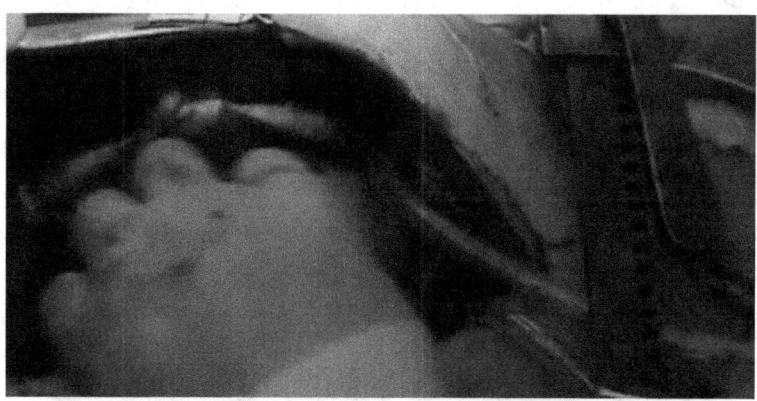

'Chest drains' tucked under bridge of retractor

Care should be taken to avoid pushing the sucker into the relatively thin-walled right atrium or right ventricle.

Having opened the chest and having accessed the heart, the resternotomy team can encounter two possible scenarios:

1) Spontaneous resumption of cardiac activity

2) No spontaneous resumption of cardiac activity

Spontaneous resumption of cardiac activity

Spontaneous resumption of cardiac activity with an appropriate output will occur most commonly in the event of tamponade. This will have occurred because of bleeding.

1) If the bleeding site is visible, it should first be digitally controlled. If the resternotomy team is appropriately experienced the 'hole' can be sutured. If this is not possible with the heart beating the need for 'going back onto cardiopulmonary bypass' should be considered to allow for safe and accurate stitch placement.

2) If the bleeding site is NOT visible i.e. there is considerable bleeding from the back of the heart it is necessary to 'go back onto cardiopulmonary bypass' to allow for finding the bleeding point and safe and accurate stitch placement to correct it.

If there is no obvious bleeding point and with the chest open, there should be further investigation (including trans-oesophageal echocardiography (TOE) and coronary angiography (if the initial operation had a coronary bypass component to it).

No spontaneous resumption of cardiac activity

At this point bimanual internal cardiac massage (ICM) should be started. This can only be performed effectively from the patient's right side.

1) **Place hands for ICM**

   Ensure the right hand is placed 'running down' the diaphragm (thus missing any inferiorly placed coronary artery bypass grafts). The right hand thus 'cups' the heart from behind. Ensure the left hand is placed over the right ventricle, avoiding the left internal mammary artery (LIMA) graft , if there is one.

2) **Gently pull up the heart slightly with the right hand** (taking tension off the LIMA) but NOT doing so if a mitral valve procedure has been done.

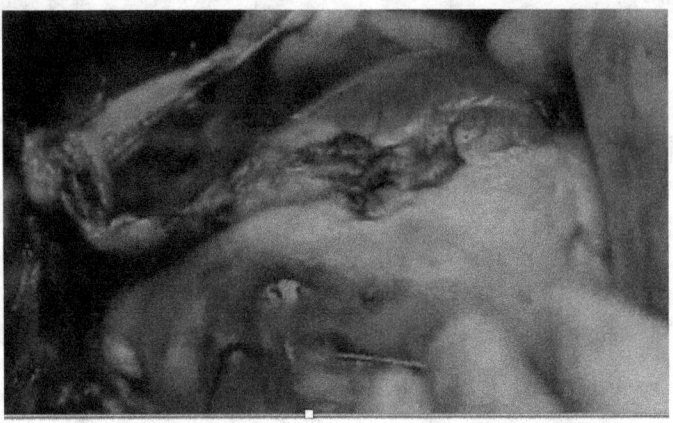

Heart being lifted by right hand relieving tension on LIMA

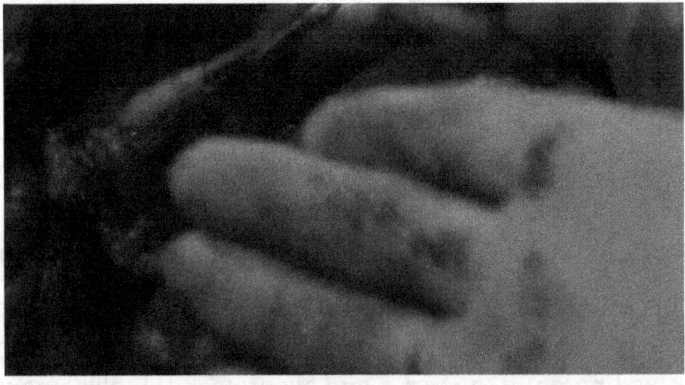

Left hand over the RV avoiding damage to LIMA

3) **Start ICM and aim for a rate of 40 – 60 compressions / minute.** The operator should also aim for a systolic blood pressure of 60 -80 mmHg.

ICM should be performed for 2 minutes. At this point ICM should be paused to allow for reassessment of the cardiac rhythm.

At this point, there are two potential rhythms:

      1)   Shockable – VF, VT

      2)   Asystole

Shockable rhythm

1)   3 x back-to-back 20J shocks

     a.   Internal defibrillation paddles placed in the position of the hands where ICM had been performed

     b.   There is no need to 'stand clear'

     c.   The paddles should be left in place during the 3 stacked shocks

2)   If no return to rhythm with output, recommence ICM and prepare for reinitiation of cardiopulmonary bypass if appropriate

3)   If return of rhythm with output consider IABP, VA ECMO, etc, and continue investigating the cause of the asystole

Non- shockable rhythm

1)   Put in two new RV pacing wires and attempt to pace VVI

2)   If no output, adrenaline (0.5 mg) can be injected into the root of the aorta

3)   If no return to output, recommence ICM and prepare for reinitiation of cardiopulmonary bypass if appropriate

4)   If output is restored, consider IABP, VA ECMO, etc, and continue investigating the cause of the asystole

In both of these scenarios, the appropriateness of continuing resuscitation needs to be a multidisciplinary decision taking into account the views of the initial operating surgeon, the intensivist and the anaesthetist involved in the patient care.

Flow Chart for Non-Return of Spontaneous Circulation (ROSC)

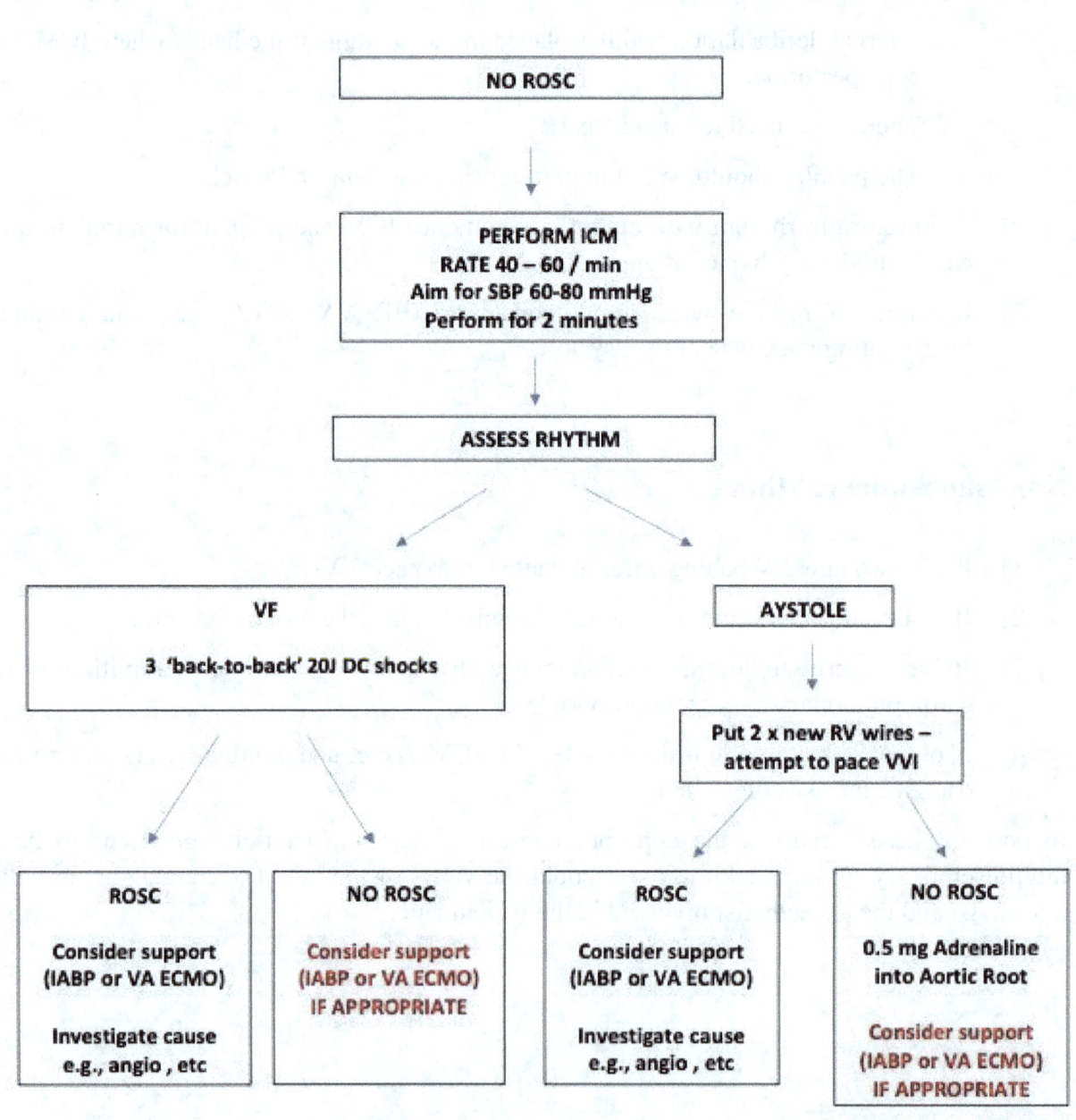

NO ROSC

↓

PERFORM ICM
RATE 40 – 60 / min
Aim for SBP 60-80 mmHg
Perform for 2 minutes

↓

ASSESS RHYTHM

VF

3 'back-to-back' 20J DC shocks

AYSTOLE

↓

Put 2 x new RV wires –
attempt to pace VVI

ROSC

Consider support
(IABP or VA ECMO)

Investigate cause
e.g., angio , etc

NO ROSC

Consider support
(IABP or VA ECMO)
IF APPROPRIATE

ROSC

Consider support
(IABP or VA ECMO)

Investigate cause
e.g., angio , etc

NO ROSC

0.5 mg Adrenaline
into Aortic Root

Consider support
(IABP or VA ECMO)
IF APPROPRIATE